Medical Terminology Suffixes Quiz

Alexander McRose

Dedication

To R.I. who motivates and comforts me.

Introduction

You know that medical terminology can be quite tricky, and that the Latinate suffixes may have several different meanings, or that they may seem similar, while, in fact, they refer to completely different concepts. This proves to be a challenge for anyone who aims to become an expert in the medical field.

Are you certain that you know everything about medical terminology suffixes?

Are you ready to prove this?

The medical terminology suffixes quiz will test your current knowledge of this subject. The point of this quiz is to give you some idea where you stand and what areas you need to focus on to pass the real exam.

Medical Terminology Suffixes Quiz Book with 240 questions and answers is a must-have for medical students, postgraduates, practitioners, nurses, medical assistants, and healthcare professionals all over the world!

Are you ready to start?

Good luck!

Quiz Instructions

1. The book contains 4 chapters with 60 questons each. Each of the four chapters is divided into four rounds of fifteen questions.

2. We recommend that you download, open, and print out the answer form, which is to be found at the end of the book. This will make the whole procedure much easier, as you won't have to write down the answers in separate columns on your own.

3. For each multiple choice question, you should read the question and circle the correct answer in the answer form.

4. After each round of questions, the correct answers are provided. You can choose whether you would like to see the correct answers immediately after having completed the round, or you can do the whole test and check all the 240 answers.

Table of Contents

CHAPTER 1 - WHAT DOES THE SUFFIX REFER TO?.............1

Chapter 1 - Round 1 Questions...2

Chapter 1 - Round 1 Correct Answer Sheet 5

Chapter 1 - Round 2 Questions...6

Chapter 1 - Round 2 Correct Answer Sheet 9

Chapter 1 - Round 3 Questions...10

Chapter 1 - Round 3 Correct Answer Sheet 13

Chapter 1 - Round 4 Questions...14

Chapter 1 - Round 4 Correct Answer Sheet 17

CHAPTER 2 - MEANING OF THE SUFFIX 18

Chapter 2 - Round 1 Questions...19

Chapter 2 - Round 1 Correct Answer Sheet 22

Chapter 2 - Round 2 Questions...23

Chapter 2 - Round 2 Correct Answer Sheet 26

Chapter 2 - Round 3 Questions...27

Chapter 2 - Round 3 Correct Answer Sheet 30

Chapter 2 - Round 4 Questions...31

Chapter 2 - Round 4 Correct Answer Sheet 34

CHAPTER 3 - WHAT DOES THE SUFFIX MEAN?...................35

Chapter 3 - Round 1 Questions...36

Chapter 3 - Round 1 Correct Answer Sheet 39

Chapter 3 - Round 2 Questions...40

Chapter 3 - Round 2 Correct Answer Sheet 43

Chapter 3 - Round 3 Questions...44

Chapter 3 - Round 3 Correct Answer Sheet 47

Chapter 3 - Round 4 Questions...48

Chapter 3 - Round 4 Correct Answer Sheet 51

CHAPTER 4 - TRUE OR FALSE **52**

Chapter 4 - Round 1 Questions...53

Chapter 4 - Round 1 Correct Answer Sheet 55

Chapter 4 - Round 2 Questions...56

Chapter 4 - Round 2 Correct Answer Sheet 58

Chapter 4 - Round 3 Questions...59

Chapter 4 - Round 3 Correct Answer Sheet 61

Chapter 4 - Round 4 Questions...62

Chapter 4 - Round 4 Correct Answer Sheet 64

ANSWER FORM **65**

Final Words 74

CHAPTER 1 - What Does the Suffix Refer To?

Chapter 1 - Round 1 Questions

1. The suffix which refers to a rupture is:

A. -graphy
B. -rrhexis
C. -penia
D. -spadias

2. The suffix which refers to paralysis is:

A. -plasia
B. -plasty
C. -plegia
D. -osis

3. The suffix which refers.to surgical suturing is:

A. -emesis
B. -geusia
C. -rrhaphy
D. -pathy

4. The suffix which refers to a process is:

A. -ation
B. -algia
C. -emia
D. -phobia

5. The suffix which refers to binding is:

A. -rupt
B. -bind
C. -pesis
D. -desis

6. The suffix which refers to producing is:

A. -fenic
B. -genic
C. -penic
D. -denic

7. The suffix which refers to the process of recording is:

A. -reco
B. -proc
C. -graphy
D. -gram

8. The suffix which refers to tissue is:

A. -ium
B. -lum
C. -aum
D. -sum

9. The suffix which refers to the process of measuring is:

A. -graph
B. -graphy
C. -meter
D. -metry

10. The suffix which refers to feeding on is:

A. -phalo
B. -phagy
C. -phasi
D. -phady

11. The suffix which refers to a rapid flow of blood is:

A. -rrhago
B. -rrhagia
C. -ectasia
D. -emia

12. The suffix which refers to a fissure is:

A. -spadias
B. -malacia
C. -geusia
D. -dipsia

13. The suffix which refers to the act of cutting or incision is:

A. -gnosis
B. -rrhagia
C. -rrhexis
D. -tomy

14. The suffix which refers to pain is:

A. -spadias
B. -algia
C. -ismus
D. -dipsia

15. The suffix which refers to thirst is:

A. -poiesis
B. -oma
C. -dipsia
D. -tome

Chapter 1 - Round 1 Correct Answer Sheet

1. B

2. C

3. C

4. A

5. D

6. B

7. C

8. A

9. D

10. B

11. B

12. A

13. D

14. B

15. C

Chapter 1 - Round 2 Questions

16. The suffix which refers to surgical operation is:

A. -ectomy
B. -operatio
C. -plasty
D. -surgy

17. The suffix which refers to blood condition is:

A. -ium
B. -emia
C. -pepsia
D. -stomy

18. The suffix which refers to a cell is

A. -cis
B. -rrhea
C. -cyte
D. -icle

19. The suffix which refers to an instrument used to record data or picture is:

A. -graph
B. -meter
C. -metry
D. -gram

20. The suffix which refers to inflammation is:

A. -infla
B. -lysis
C. -osis
D. -itis

21. The suffix which refers to a disease or disorder is:

A. -paresis
B. -pathy
C. -pexy
D. -plasty

22. The suffix which refers to exaggerated fear or sensitivity is:

A. -rupt
B. -tomy
C. -phobia
D. -trophy

23. The suffix which refers to falling or drooping is:

A. -ptosis
B. -ptysis
C. -ptisis
D. -osis

24. The suffix which refers to hardening is:

A. -plasia
B. -rrhexis
C. -sclerosis
D. -spadias

25. The suffix which refers to a cutting instrument is:

A. -come
B. -nome
C. -tome
D. -gome

26. The suffix which refers to enzyme is:

A. -ise
B. -ose
C. -asy
D. -ase

27. The suffix which refers to secreting is:

A. -crine
B. -drine
C. -prine
D. -pathy

28. The suffix which refers to taste is:

A. -lusia
B. -erusia
C. -sclerosis
D. -geusia

29. The suffix which refers to treatment is:

A. -stomy
B. -ics
C. -penia
D. -ips

30. The suffix which refers to softening is:

A. -malacia
B. -falacia
C. -dalacia
D. -nalacia

Chapter 1 - Round 2 Correct Answer Sheet

16. A

17. B

18. C

19. A

20. D

21. B

22. C

23.A

24. C

25. C

26. D

27. A

28. D

29. B

30. A

Chapter 1 - Round 3 Questions

31. The suffix which refers to hernia is:

A. -dele
B. -cele
C. -bele
D. -nia

32. The suffix which refers to vomiting condition is:

A. -malacia
B. -sclerosis
C. -emesis
D. -algia

33. The suffix which refers to a record or picture is:

A. -gram
B. -ium
C. -lysis
D. -metry

34. The suffix which refers to an instrument used to measure or count is:

A. -metry
B. -meter
C. -graph
D. -graphy

35. The suffix which refers to conditions related to eating is:

A. -gia
B. -lagia
C. -algia
D. -phagia

36. The suffix which refers to a formation or development is:

A. -blasia
B. -dasia
C. -clasia
D. -plasia

37. The suffix which refers to breaking or bursting is:

A. -supt
B. -pupt
C. -rupt
D. -cupt

38. The suffix which refers to the creation of an opening is:

A. -omy
B. -crom
C. -nomy
D. -stomy

39. The suffix which refers to turning is:

A. -sion
B. -iatry
C. -version
D. -oma

40. The suffix which refers to destroying is:

A. -cidal
B. -fidal
C. -nidal
D. -didal

41. The suffix which refers to a field in medicine is:

A. -etry
B. -iatry
C. -itry
D. -otry

42. The suffix which refers to destruction or separation is:

A. -phagia
B. -lysis
C. -genic
D. -cele

43. The suffix which refers to deficiency is:

A. -penia
B. -asthenia
C. -ectasia
D. -malacia

44. The suffix which refers to production is:

A. -ptosis
B. -ptysis
C. -poiesis
D. -phobia

45. The suffix which refers to the use of an instrument for viewing is:

A. -opy
B. -scopy
C. -ics
D. -emia

Chapter 1 - Round 3 Correct Answer Sheet

31. B

32. C

33. A

34. B

35. D

36. D

37. C

38. D

39. C

40. A

41. B

42. B

43. A

44. C

45. B

Chapter 1 - Round 4 Questions

46. The suffix which refers to a condition, disease or increase is:

A. -acusis
B. -ation
C. -cyte
D. -osis

47. The suffix which refers to spitting is:

A. -geusia
B. -iatry
C. -ptysis
D. -ectasia

48. The suffix which refers to dripping or trickling is:

A. -staxis
B. -lepsy
C. -plegia
D. -stomy

49. The suffix which refers to crushing is:

A. -pathy
B. -tripsy
C. -phagy
D. -osis

50. The suffix which refers to hearing is:

A. -rrhexis
B. -rrhea
C. -rrhaphy
D. -acusis

51. The suffix which refers to something small is:

A. -icle
B. -ium
C. -ice
D. -ics

52. The suffix which refers to digestion or the digestive tract is:

A. -plegia
B. -plexy
C. -pepsia
D. -plasia

53. The suffix which refers to an instrument for viewing is:

A. -scopy
B. -scope
C. -ectasia
D. -stomy

54. The suffix which refers to weakness is:

A. -lepsy
B. -pepsy
C. -opsy
D. -asthenia

55. The suffix which refers to a tumor or mass is:

A. -oma
B. -stoma
C. -ema
D. -stomy

56. The suffix which refers to contraction is:

A. -sis
B. -amalis
C. -stalsis
D. -analis

57. The suffix which refers to bursting is:

A. -phagy
B. -rrhage
C. -bragy
D. -brage

58. The suffix which refers to knowledge is:

A. -opsis
B. -ptysis
C. -ptosis
D. -gnosis

59. The suffix which refers to a slight paralysis is:

A. -paresis
B. -stalsis
C. -stasis
D. -paris

60. The suffix which refers to pressure is:

A. -oma
B. -dipsia
C. -pathy
D. -tension

Chapter 1 - Round 4 Correct Answer Sheet

46. D

47. C

48. A

49. B

50. D

51. A

52. C

53. B

54. D

55. A

56. C

57. B

58. D

59. A

60. D

CHAPTER 2 - Meaning of the Suffix

Chapter 2 - Round 1 Questions

1. The suffix meaning killing is:

A. -edal
B. -cidal
C. -adal
D. -odal

2. The suffix meaning deficiency is:

A. -denia
B. -menia
C. -penia
D. -cenia

3. The suffix meaning development is:

A. -asia
B. -masia
C. -plasia
D. -ole

4. The suffix meaning downward placement is:

A. -ptosis
B. -file
C. -sis
D. -dis

5. The suffix meaning hardening is:

A. -geusia
B. -lysis
C. -penia
D. -sclerosis

6. The suffix meaning creation of an opening is:

A. -trophy
B. -stomy
C. -tome
D. -nomy

7. The suffix meaning nourishment is:

A. -nuri
B. -poiesis
C. -trophy
D. -metry

8. The suffix meaning expansion is:

A. -ectasia
B. -phago
C. -lepsis
D. -sion

9. The suffix meaning pouching is:

A. -dele
B. -mele
C. -bele
D. -cele

10. The suffix meaning pain is:

A. -dunia
B. -dynia
C. -dania
D. -mania

11. The suffix meaning record or picture is:

A. -cram
B. -gram
C. -dram
D. -eram

12. The suffix meaning one who specializes in is:

A. -ist
B. -ost
C. -ast
D. -be

13. The suffix meaning resemblance to is:

A. -old
B. -aid
C. -ance
D. -oid

14. The suffix meaning digestive tract is:

A. -act
B. -pepsia
C. -digest
D. -gest

15. The suffix meaning spitting is:

A. -lepsis
B. -poiesis
C. -ptysis
D. -sclerosis

Chapter 2 - Round 1 Correct Answer Sheet

1. B

2. C

3. C

4. A

5. D

6. B

7. C

8. A

9. D

10. B

11. B

12. A

13. D

14. B

15. C

Chapter 2 - Round 2 Questions

16. The suffix meaning paralysis is:

A. -plegia
B. -malacia
C. -phobia
D. -geusia

17. The suffix meaning fissure is:

A. -ectasis
B. -spadias
C. -rrhaphy
D. -pathy

18. The suffix meaning crushing is:

A. -ist
B. -itis
C. -tripsy
D. -ium

19. The suffix meaning toward or in the direction of is:

A. -ad
B. -ed
C. -od
D. -id

20. The suffix meaning thirst is:

A. -pepsia
B. -spadias
C. -staxis
D. -dipsia

21. The suffix meaning formative is:

A. -osis
B. -genic
C. -acal
D. -ase

22. The suffix meaning process of recording is:

A. -ectomy
B. -itis
C. -graphy
D. -graph

23. The suffix meaning inflammation is:

A. -itis
B. -ismus
C. -lysis
D. -oma

24. The suffix meaning destruction is:

A. -itis
B. -logy
C. -lysis
D. -phagia

25. The suffix meaning disorder is:

A. -geusia
B. -centesis
C. -pathy
D. -ula

26. The suffix meaning exaggerated fear is:

A. -oma
B. -oid
C. -stalsis
D. -phobia

27. The suffix meaning break is:

A. -rupt
B. -pathy
C. -gnosis
D. -ation

28. The suffix meaning cutting instrument is:

A. -ment
B. -ame
C. -omy
D. -tome

29. The suffix meaning reconstruction is:

A. -tion
B. -plasty
C. -ismus
D. -ectasia

30. The suffix meaning cell is:

A. -cyte
B. -phago
C. -phagy
D. -ptysis

Chapter 2 - Round 2 Correct Answer Sheet

16. A

17. B

18. C

19. A

20. D

21. B

22. C

23. A

24. C

25. C

26. D

27. A

28. D

29. B

30. A

Chapter 2 - Round 3 Questions

31. The suffix meaning abnormal narrowing is:

A. -centesis
B. -stenosis
C. -stecesis
D. -centosis

32. The suffix meaning destroying is:

A. -vide
B. -zide
C. -cide
D. -cidy

33. The suffix meaning having the form of is:

A. -form
B. -fore
C. -fora
D. -fori

34. The suffix meaning treatment is:

A. -ment
B. -ics
C. -menis
D. -ritis

35. The suffix meaning softening is:

A. -dacia
B. -cia
C. -bia
D. -malacia

36. The suffix meaning fixation is:

A. -tion
B. -fixa
C. -texy
D. -pexy

37. The suffix meaning surgical suturing is:

A. -rrhexis
B. -ript
C. -rrhaphy
D. -rupt

38. The suffix meaning cell is:

A. -ryte
B. -cite
C. -rite
D. -cyte

39. The suffix meaning knowledge is:

A. -osis
B. asis
C. -gnosis
D. -sis

40. The suffix meaning the nature of is:

A. -ite
B. -turo
C. -ture
D. -ato

41. The suffix meaning increase is:

A. -esis
B. -osis
C. -isis
D. -asis

42. The suffix meaning dilation is:

A. -sis
B. -ectasis
C. -octo
D. -nuno

43. The suffix meaning contraction is:

A. -ismus
B. -paresis
C. -ptosis
D. -tripsy

44. The suffix meaning slight paralysis is:

A. -pathy
B. -phagy
C. -paresis
D. -phago

45. The suffix meaning small is:

A. -oid
B. -icle
C. -oma
D. -ama

Chapter 2 - Round 3 Correct Answer Sheet

31. B

32. C

33. A

34. B

35. D

36. D

37. C

38. D

39. C

40. A

41. B

42. B

43. A

44. C

45. B

Chapter 2 - Round 4 Questions

46. The suffix meaning tissue is:

A. -dum
B. -bum
C. -cum
D. -ium

47. The suffix meaning use of instrument for viewing is:

A. -ectomy
B. -ation
C. -scopy
D. -asthenia

48. The suffix meaning binding is:

A. -desis
B. -ismus
C. -lysis
D. -pepsia

49. The suffix meaning disease is:

A. -metry
B. -ism
C. -penia
D. -scopy

50. The suffix meaning mass is:

A. -ula
B. -idi
C. -ema
D. -oma

51. The suffix meaning production is:

A. -poiesis
B. -emesis
C. -gnosis
D. -poiesis

52. The suffix meaning body part removal is:

A. -plexy
B. -tomy
C. -ectomy
D. -rrhagia

53. The suffix meaning the study of is:

A. -or
B. -logy
C. -penia
D. -cyte

54. The suffix meaning feeding on is:

A. -cele
B. -pexy
C. -osis
D. -phagy

55. The suffix meaning contraction is:

A. -stalsis
B. -tion
C. -sis
D. -asis

56. The suffix meaning turning is:

A. -sion
B. -itis
C. -version
D. -rupt

57. The suffix meaning surgical puncture is:

A. -desis
B. -centesis
C. -pepsia
D. -phobia

58. The suffix meaning weakness is:

A. -dipsia
B. -dynia
C. -geusia
D. -asthenia

59. The suffix meaning taste is:

A. -geusia
B. -ismus
C. -desis
D. -desus

60. The suffix meaning ingestion is:

A. -ilo
B. -ion
C. -alo
D. -phagia

Chapter 2 - Round 4 Correct Answer Sheet

46. D

47. C

48. A

49. B

50. D

51. A

52. C

53. B

54. D

55. A

56. C

57. B

58. D

59. A

60. D

CHAPTER 3 - What Does the Suffix Mean?

Chapter 3 - Round 1 Questions

1. The suffix -centesis means:

A. discharge
B. surgical puncture
C. fixation
D. attraction for

2. The suffix -dipsia means:

A. enzyme
B. hearing
C. thirst
D. process

3. The suffix -emesis means:

A. knowledge
B. reconstruction
C. vomiting condition
D. stroke

4. The suffix -ectasis means:

A. dilation
B. attack
C. deficiency
D. from

5. The suffix -geusia means:

A. pertaining to
B. rupture
C. softening
D. taste

6. The suffix -itis means:

A. blood condition
B. inflammation
C. contraction
D. fluid collection

7. The suffix -oid means:

A. having the form of
B. instrument used to measure or count
C. resemblance to
D. instrument for viewing

8. The suffix -plasia means:

A. formation
B. cell
C. falling
D. fixation

9. The suffix -rrhagia means:

A. removal of a body part
B. use of instrument for viewing
C. vomiting condition
D. rapid flow of blood

10. The suffix -scopy means:

A. pertaining to
B. use of instrument for viewing
C. disease
D. discharge

11. The suffix -tension means:

A. paralysis
B. pressure
C. dripping
D. crushing

12. The suffix -ula means:

A. small
B. big
C. binding
D. development

13. The suffix -cidal means:

A. inflammation
B. incision
C. having the form of
D. killing

14. The suffix -emesis means:

A. fixation
B. vomiting condition
C. reconstruction
D. pressure

15. The suffix -gnosis means:

A. discharge
B. stroke
C. knowledge
D. surgical puncture

Chapter 3 - Round 1 Correct Answer Sheet

1. B

2. C

3. C

4. A

5. D

6. B

7. C

8. A

9. D

10. B

11. B

12. A

13. D

14. B

15. C

Chapter 3 - Round 2 Questions

16. The suffix -ite means:

A. the nature of
B. instrument for viewing
C. nothing
D. reconstruction

17. The suffix -malacia means:

A. incision
B. softening
C. dilation
D. cutting instrument

18. The suffix -penia means:

A. enzyme
B. from
C. deficiency
D. paralysis

19. The suffix -ptosis means:

A. falling
B. sensitivity
C. stopping
D. weakness

20. The suffix -rupt means:

A. nothing
B. rupture
C. spasm
D. burst

21. The suffix -staxis means:

A. academic study
B. dripping
C. burst forth
D. deficiency

22. The suffix -tripsy means:

A. fluid collection
B. pain
C. crushing
D. rapid flow of blood

23. The suffix -crine means:

A. to secrete
B. fixation
C. paralysis
D. sensitivity

24. The suffix -ectomy means:

A. spasm
B. spitting
C. removal of a body part
D. nothing

25. The suffix -graphy means:

A. process of measuring
B. instrument for viewing
C. process of recording
D. process of listening

26. The suffix -lepsy means:

A. rupture
B. structure
C. the nature of
D. seizure

27. The suffix -oma means:

A. fluid collection
B. to secrete
C. vomiting condition
D. spitting

28. The suffix -poiesis means:

A. crushing
B. creation of an opening
C. having the form of
D. production

29. The suffix -trophy means:

A. fixation
B. development
C. slight paralysis
D. spasm

30. The suffix -acusis means:

A. hearing
B. incision
C. destruction
D. disease

Chapter 3 - Round 2 Correct Answer Sheet

16. A

17. B

18. C

19. A

20. D

21. B

22. C

23. A

24. C

25. C

26. D

27. A

28. D

29. B

30. A

Chapter 3 - Round 3 Questions

31. The suffix -ation means:

A. dilation
B. process
C. discharge
D. dripping

32. The suffix -ectasia means:

A. hardening
B. softening
C. expansion
D. nothing

33. The suffix -genic means:

A. producing
B. thirst
C. dripping
D. blood condition

34. The suffix -ium means:

A. cell
B. structure
C. contraction
D. falling

35. The suffix -metry means:

A. process of recording
B. rapid flow of blood
C. removal of a body part
D. process of measuring

36. The suffix -philia means:

A. spasm
B. to secrete
C. nothing
D. attraction for

37. The suffix -ptysis means:

A. slit
B. sleeping
C. spitting
D. walking

38. The suffix -rrhea means:

A. seizure
B. inflammation
C. incision
D. discharge

39. The suffix -stenosis means:

A. killing
B. process of measuring
C. abnormal narrowing in a blood vessel
D. slight paralysis

40. The suffix -tome means:

A. cutting instrument
B. walking
C. development
D. binding

41. The suffix -emia means:

A. burst
B. blood condition
C. crushing
D. fixation

42. The suffix -ismus means:

A. sleeping
B. spasm
C. softening
D. stroke

43. The suffix -paresis means:

A. slight paralysis
B. sensitivity
C. paralysis
D. knowledge

44. The suffix -plegia means:

A. discharge
B. slight paralysis
C. paralysis
D. hernia

45. The suffix -sclerosis means:

A. nothing
B. hardening
C. incision
D. sleeping

Chapter 3 - Round 3 Correct Answer Sheet

31. B

32. C

33. A

34. B

35. D

36. D

37. C

38. D

39. C

40. A

41. B

42. B

43. A

44. C

45. B

Chapter 3 - Round 4 Questions

46. The suffix -scope means:

A. walking
B. burst forth
C. attack
D. instrument for viewing

47. The suffix -stomy means:

A. discharge
B. cutting
C. creation of an opening
D. cutting instrument

48. The suffix -cele means:

A. hernia
B. fixation
C. incision
D. cell

49. The suffix -dynia means:

A. nothing
B. pain
C. dilation
D. deficiency

50. The suffix -ism means:

A. incision
B. inflammation
C. information
D. disease

51. The suffix -or means:

A. one who
B. before
C. after
D. now

52. The suffix -plasty means:

A. plastic
B. producing
C. reconstruction
D. sensitivity

53. The suffix -spadias means:

A. nothing
B. slit
C. slight paralysis
D. sleeping

54. The suffix -tomy means:

A. surgical puncture
B. surgical suturing
C. toward
D. incision

55. The suffix -asthenia means:

A. weakness
B. taste
C. producing
D. reconstruction

56. The suffix -gen means:

A. removal of a body part
B. above
C. from
D. below

57. The suffix -lysis means:

A. creation of an opening
B. destruction
C. one who
D. organized knowledge

58. The suffix -pexy means:

A. down
B. under
C. walking
D. fixation

59. The suffix -plexy means:

A. stroke
B. left
C. right
D. to secrete

60. The suffix -stalsis means:

A. weakness
B. attack
C. nothing
D. contraction

Chapter 3 - Round 4 Correct Answer Sheet

46. D

47. C

48. A

49. B

50. D

51. A

52. C

53. B

54. D

55. A

56. C

57. B

58. D

59. A

60. D

Chapter 4 - True or False

Chapter 4 - Round 1 Questions

1. The suffix -cele means hernia

A. True
B. False

2. The suffix -ectasis means fluid collection

A. True
B. False

3. The suffix -genic means spitting

A. True
B. False

4. The suffix -ite means the nature of

A. True
B. False

5. The suffix -lysis means destruction

A. True
B. False

6. The suffix -osis means hardening

A. True
B. False

7. The suffix -plegia means paralysis

A. True
B. False

8. The suffix -rrhaphy means surgical suturing

A. True
B. False

9. The suffix -scopy means removal of a body part

A. True
B. False

10. The suffix -tome means cutting instrument

A. True
B. False

11. The suffix -ula means big

A. True
B. False

12. The suffix -crine means to secrete

A. True
B. False

13. The suffix -form means organized knowledge

A. True
B. False

14. The suffix -ics means organized knowledge

A. True
B. False

15. The suffix -lepsy means pressure

A. True
B. False

Chapter 4 - Round 1 Correct Answer Sheet

1. A

2. B

3. B

4. A

5. A

6. B

7. A

8. A

9. B

10. A

11. B

12. A

13. B

14. A

15. B

Chapter 4 - Round 2 Questions

16. The suffix -phobia means attraction for

A. True
B. False

17. The suffix -ismus means spasm

A. True
B. False

18. The suffix -plexy means falling

A. True
B. False

19. The suffix -centesis means surgical puncture

A. True
B. False

20. The suffix -algia means cell

A. True
B. False

21. The suffix -gen means from

A. True
B. False

22. The suffix -ism means disease

A. True
B. False

23. The suffix -logy means seizure

A. True
B. False

24. The suffix -or means toward

A. True
B. False

25. The suffix -plasty means reconstruction

A. True
B. False

26. The suffix -rrhage means slight paralysis

A. True
B. False

27. The suffix -sclerosis means discharge

A. True
B. False

28. The suffix -tension means pressure

A. True
B. False

29. The suffix -cidal means killing

A. True
B. False

30. The suffix -ectasia means expansion

A. True
B. False

Chapter 4 - Round 2 Correct Answer Sheet

16. B

17. A

18. B

19. A

20. B

21. A

22. A

23. B

24. B

25. A

26. B

27. B

28. A

29. A

30. A

Chapter 4 - Round 3 Questions

31. The suffix -malacia means inflammation

A. True
B. False

32. The suffix -oma means fluid collection

A. True
B. False

33. The suffix -plasia means dilation

A. True
B. False

34. The suffix -rupt means burst

A. True
B. False

35. The suffix -staxis means dripping

A. True
B. False

36. The suffix -trophy means attraction for

A. True
B. False

37. The suffix -asthenia means producing

A. True
B. False

38. The suffix -dipsia means thirst

A. True
B. False

39. The suffix -itis means inflammation

A. True
B. False

40. The suffix -paresis means slight paralysis

A. True
B. False

41. The suffix -ptosis means dripping

A. True
B. False

42. The suffix -rrhexis means spasm

A. True
B. False

43. The suffix -stenosis means abnormal narrowing in a blood vessel

A. True
B. False

44. The suffix -emesis means sensitivity

A. True
B. False

45. The suffix -lepsis means attack

A. True
B. False

Chapter 4 - Round 3 Correct Answer Sheet

31. B

32. A

33. B

34. A

35. A

36. B

37. B

38. A

39. A

40. A

41. B

42. B

43. A

44. B

45. A

Chapter 4 - Round 4 Questions

46. The suffix -desis means incision

A. True
B. False

47. The suffix -geusia means taste

A. True
B. False

48. The suffix -ium means structure

A. True
B. False

49. The suffix -oid means process of measuring

A. True
B. False

50. The suffix -philia means attraction for

A. True
B. False

51. The suffix -rrhagia means rapid flow of blood

A. True
B. False

52. The suffix -stalsis means to secrete

A. True
B. False

53. The suffix -tripsy means crushing

A. True
B. False

54. The suffix -ectomy means attraction for

A. True
B. False

55. The suffix -acusis means hearing

A. True
B. False

56. The suffix -emia means expansion

A. True
B. False

57. The suffix -ad means toward

A. True
B. False

58. The suffix -gnosis means knowledge

A. True
B. False

59. The suffix -penia means discharge

A. True
B. False

60. The suffix -ation means process

A. True
B. False

Chapter 4 - Round 4 Correct Answer Sheet

46. B

47. A

48. A

49. B

50. A

51. A

52. B

53. A

54. B

55. A

56. B

57. A

58. A

59. B

60. A

Answer Form

Chapter 1 - What does the suffix refer to?

Round 1 Questions

1.	A	B	C	D
2.	A	B	C	D
3.	A	B	C	D
4.	A	B	C	D
5.	A	B	C	D
6.	A	B	C	D
7.	A	B	C	D
8.	A	B	C	D
9.	A	B	C	D
10.	A	B	C	D
11.	A	B	C	D
12.	A	B	C	D
13.	A	B	C	D
14.	A	B	C	D
15.	A	B	C	D

Round 2 Questions

16.	A	B	C	D
17.	A	B	C	D
18.	A	B	C	D
19.	A	B	C	D
20.	A	B	C	D
21.	A	B	C	D
22.	A	B	C	D
23.	A	B	C	D
24.	A	B	C	D
25.	A	B	C	D
26.	A	B	C	D
27.	A	B	C	D
28.	A	B	C	D
29.	A	B	C	D
30.	A	B	C	D

Round 3 Questions

31.	A	B	C	D
32.	A	B	C	D
33.	A	B	C	D
34.	A	B	C	D
35.	A	B	C	D
36.	A	B	C	D
37.	A	B	C	D
38.	A	B	C	D
39.	A	B	C	D
40.	A	B	C	D
41.	A	B	C	D
42.	A	B	C	D
43.	A	B	C	D
44.	A	B	C	D
45.	A	B	C	D

Round 4 Questions

46.	A	B	C	D
47.	A	B	C	D
48.	A	B	C	D
49.	A	B	C	D
50.	A	B	C	D
51.	A	B	C	D
52.	A	B	C	D
53.	A	B	C	D
54.	A	B	C	D
55.	A	B	C	D
56.	A	B	C	D
57.	A	B	C	D
58.	A	B	C	D
59.	A	B	C	D
60.	A	B	C	D

Chapter 2 - Recognize the meaning of the suffix

Round 1 Questions

1.	A	B	C	D
2.	A	B	C	D
3.	A	B	C	D
4.	A	B	C	D
5.	A	B	C	D
6.	A	B	C	D
7.	A	B	C	D
8.	A	B	C	D
9.	A	B	C	D
10.	A	B	C	D
11.	A	B	C	D
12.	A	B	C	D
13.	A	B	C	D
14.	A	B	C	D
15.	A	B	C	D

Round 2 Questions

16.	A	B	C	D
17.	A	B	C	D
18.	A	B	C	D
19.	A	B	C	D
20.	A	B	C	D
21.	A	B	C	D
22.	A	B	C	D
23.	A	B	C	D
24.	A	B	C	D
25.	A	B	C	D
26.	A	B	C	D
27.	A	B	C	D
28.	A	B	C	D
29.	A	B	C	D
30.	A	B	C	D

Round 3 Questions

31.	A	B	C	D
32.	A	B	C	D
33.	A	B	C	D
34.	A	B	C	D
35.	A	B	C	D
36.	A	B	C	D
37.	A	B	C	D
38.	A	B	C	D
39.	A	B	C	D
40.	A	B	C	D
41.	A	B	C	D
42.	A	B	C	D
43.	A	B	C	D
44.	A	B	C	D
45.	A	B	C	D

Round 4 Questions

46.	A	B	C	D
47.	A	B	C	D
48.	A	B	C	D
49.	A	B	C	D
50.	A	B	C	D
51.	A	B	C	D
52.	A	B	C	D
53.	A	B	C	D
54.	A	B	C	D
55.	A	B	C	D
56.	A	B	C	D
57.	A	B	C	D
58.	A	B	C	D
59.	A	B	C	D
60.	A	B	C	D

Chapter 3 - What does the suffix mean?

Round 1 Questions

1.	A	B	C	D
2.	A	B	C	D
3.	A	B	C	D
4.	A	B	C	D
5.	A	B	C	D
6.	A	B	C	D
7.	A	B	C	D
8.	A	B	C	D
9.	A	B	C	D
10.	A	B	C	D
11.	A	B	C	D
12.	A	B	C	D
13.	A	B	C	D
14.	A	B	C	D
15.	A	B	C	D

Round 2 Questions

16.	A	B	C	D
17.	A	B	C	D
18.	A	B	C	D
19.	A	B	C	D
20.	A	B	C	D
21.	A	B	C	D
22.	A	B	C	D
23.	A	B	C	D
24.	A	B	C	D
25.	A	B	C	D
26.	A	B	C	D
27.	A	B	C	D
28.	A	B	C	D
29.	A	B	C	D
30.	A	B	C	D

Round 3 Questions

31.	A	B	C	D
32.	A	B	C	D
33.	A	B	C	D
34.	A	B	C	D
35.	A	B	C	D
36.	A	B	C	D
37.	A	B	C	D
38.	A	B	C	D
39.	A	B	C	D
40.	A	B	C	D
41.	A	B	C	D
42.	A	B	C	D
43.	A	B	C	D
44.	A	B	C	D
45.	A	B	C	D

Round 4 Questions

46.	A	B	C	D
47.	A	B	C	D
48.	A	B	C	D
49.	A	B	C	D
50.	A	B	C	D
51.	A	B	C	D
52.	A	B	C	D
53.	A	B	C	D
54.	A	B	C	D
55.	A	B	C	D
56.	A	B	C	D
57.	A	B	C	D
58.	A	B	C	D
59.	A	B	C	D
60.	A	B	C	D

Chapter 4 - True or False

Round 1 Questions

1.	A	B
2.	A	B
3.	A	B
4.	A	B
5.	A	B
6.	A	B
7.	A	B
8.	A	B
9.	A	B
10.	A	B
11.	A	B
12.	A	B
13.	A	B
14.	A	B
15.	A	B

Round 2 Questions

16.	A	B
17.	A	B
18.	A	B
19.	A	B
20.	A	B
21.	A	B
22.	A	B
23.	A	B
24.	A	B
25.	A	B
26.	A	B
27.	A	B
28.	A	B
29.	A	B
30.	A	B

Round 3 Questions

31.	A	B
32.	A	B
33.	A	B
34.	A	B
35.	A	B
36.	A	B
37.	A	B
38.	A	B
39.	A	B
40.	A	B
41.	A	B
42.	A	B
43.	A	B
44.	A	B
45.	A	B

Round 4 Questions

46.	A	B
47.	A	B
48.	A	B
49.	A	B
50.	A	B
51.	A	B
52.	A	B
53.	A	B
54.	A	B
55.	A	B
56.	A	B
57.	A	B
58.	A	B
59.	A	B
60.	A	B

Final Words

I hope you enjoyed using this quiz book as much as I enjoyed making it. It was truly a labor of love.

I'm always striving to improve my books, and one of the ways I can do that is if I get an honest feedback on my work.

It would help me out a lot if you could leave your honest review.

Thank you so much for doing this!

Alexander McRose

Printed in Great Britain
by Amazon